30-MINUTE
FOR WEIGHT LOSS

BY AMANDA HYATT

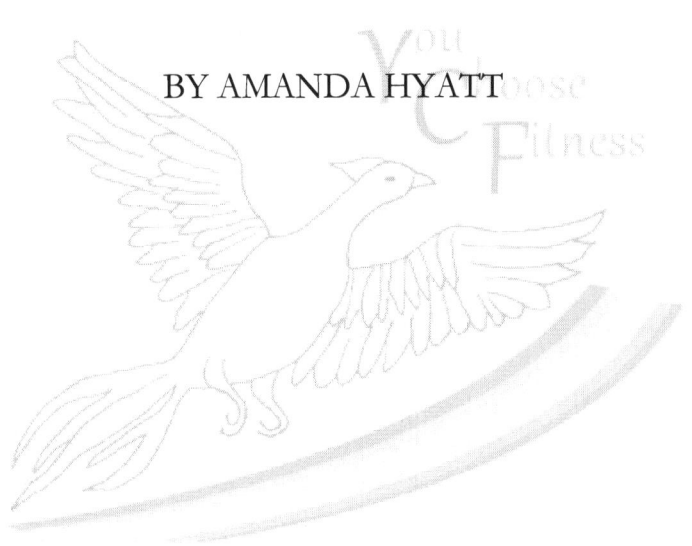

© 2015 AMANDA HYATT

No part of this book may be reproduced, stored in a retrieval system or transmitted by any means without the written permission of the author

ISBN: 978-1-326-46669-5

Find us on the web:

http://www.youchoosefitness.co.uk

On Facebook for weight loss and nutritional secrets, hints & tips:

http://www.facebook.com/groups/youchoosefitness

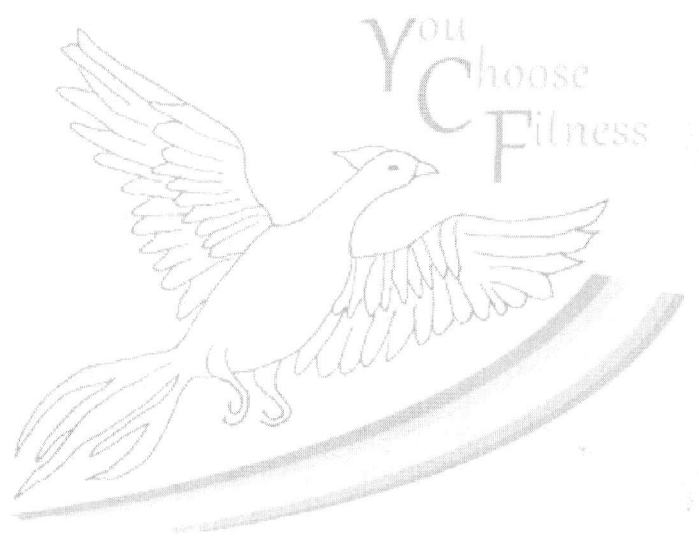

FOR THE WALKERS
AND THE DOG WALKERS

WHO WOULD LIKE THEIR WALKS TO
MAKE A DIFFERENCE

TO THEIR HEALTH
TO THEIR FITNESS
TO THEIR WEIGHT

CONTENTS

EVERY JOURNEY BEGINS WITH A SINGLE STEP 2
WHAT DO YOU MEAN BY 'WALKING WITH PURPOSE'? 5
WALKING LEVELS EXPLAINED 8
WALK ONE Starter For .... 30? 10
WALK TWO Who fartlekked? 12
WALK THREE Like clockwork 16
WALK FOUR Stepping up a gear 20
WALK FIVE Simple and effective 22
WALK SIX Tempo walk 24
WALK SEVEN How to confuse your dog 26
WALK EIGHT Further Faster Stronger 30
WALK NINE Pot luck 32
WALK TEN A little more like a workout 36
WHAT NEXT? ONE STEP FURTHER 38
5 TIPS TO ENSURE THAT EVERY WORKOUT IS A SUCCESS: ... 40
10-MINUTE WORKOUT 42
15-MINUTE WORKOUT 44
20-MINUTE WORKOUT 48
5 MOST COMMON WEIGHT LOSS ERRORS 52
5 TOP TIPS FOR WEIGHT LOSS 54
DON'T STOP THERE! 56

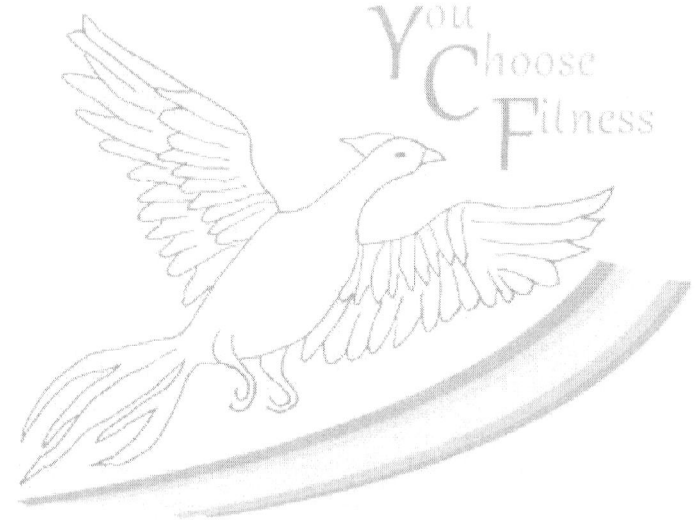

EVERY JOURNEY BEGINS WITH A SINGLE STEP

Whether it's your first step or you're a seasoned walker, thank you for your interest in *30-Minute Walks for Weight Loss* – a book that comes with my heart and soul in it, alongside the very best of wishes that you both enjoy adding a little spice to your walks *and* that they add a little variety to your weight loss journey.

I've always been an active and outdoorsy sort of person, but after Child No. 4 was dropped on my doorstep by a friendly stork I stopped making time for myself (yes, time has to be 'made'!), stopped exercising appropriately and the pounds slowly crept on. I think we can all agree that the less you do the less you feel like doing? That saying 'If you want something done, ask a busy person' is so true. As we spend more time sitting down or staying indoors, it gets harder and harder to get up off the couch and get active – or indeed to get outdoors on a regular basis.

It's this kind of 'difficulty' that the healthcare professionals recognise and why such emphasis is placed these days on that regular 30 minute walk! It is SO important. It will keep you healthy, it will boost your energy and your mood (provided you don't sabotage it all with a diet soda along the way!) and if you've barely moved in the last few weeks/months, then it's certainly the place to begin.

HOWEVER (that's a *big* however), if you're trying to lose weight then you want that walk to contribute to your weight loss as well as your health, don't you? You have two options here. You can increase the 30 minutes to a 60-minute walk – doing what you always do but extending the time … OR … you can stick to 30 minutes but incorporate real purpose into those sessions, saving you time but doubling the effectiveness. To burn that fat off your walks need purpose, intent and, even more importantly, variety. Different scenery may be great for the soul but walking at the same pace, marching along the flats, struggling with the same hills? For the body, *that* is all the same, so while the mind is continually refreshed your body is BORED and will just go to sleep.

HERE … in this little booklet … you'll find walks that will keep your body wide awake and working for you in the minimum amount of time. You can use them for dog-walking or do them pushing a buggy. All you need is a watch and for some of them you *will* need to get yourself to a hill. Otherwise, roads or fields, woodland, trails … the choice of terrain is yours. All you have to do is scribble down or memorise the walk you're planning to do on that particular day and off you go! Mix these in with 60-minute walks when you have time and you can be confident that you are not only staying healthy but ALSO burning those unwanted calories.

One more thing. Remember to smile ☺

Enjoy the journey.

WHAT DO YOU MEAN BY 'WALKING WITH PURPOSE'?

This is a vitally important question and the key to making a real difference to your walks. I'm pretty sure that if we were walking side by side right now and I turned and said 'Let's pick up the pace', you would simply walk a little faster. From now on, you need to be able to walk a little faster – and then faster again … and again!

For the walks in this book, your 'normal' walking pace (from now on known as Level 1 pace) should already be a little faster than a stroll (if strolling is what you're used to). It's also a little faster than your meander with your dog (including throwing sticks etc.). Level 1 pace, therefore, is just a little faster than you normally walk – so be sure to keep this in mind as soon as you set foot outside the door. Walking a little faster than normal is trickier than you think! I'm willing to bet that after about 3 minutes you will have already slowed back to your natural 'strolling' pace, so watch out! Think of each walk as one with purpose and that way you will be more attentive and focussed on what you're doing. It is actually quite demanding to walk at a faster pace than your 'natural' one and to sustain it! It takes concentration.

So ... we've got your 30-minute Level 1 walk pace sorted– just a little faster than usual, ok? So NOW – when you see terms Level 2 and Level 3 you *really* need to put in effort. Stand up tall, squeeze bum, pull tummy button in, shoulders back, head high, then pump those arms and really move! Your legs should be moving at double your usual speed – but without any running!! This is FAST walking and is crucial for these walks to be effective, so do be prepared for those changes of speed.

The walking 'levels' are explained on the next page. However, it is vital to clarify that when I talk about speed I'm talking about YOUR speed. Not anybody else's speed. This is YOUR walk, YOUR workout – at YOUR pace!! We all naturally walk at different speeds – according to size, age, ability and any combination of these, so please do NOT compare yourself to anyone else. Your 'fast' could be somebody else's 'natural' pace. Don't be disheartened. This is completely normal and this is not a competition. If you walk with a friend and you find yourself struggling to keep up OR stressed because they're slower than you, then save these purposeful walks for another day and keep walks with friends for pure enjoyment. This is the key to success. Your walk, your journey, your way.

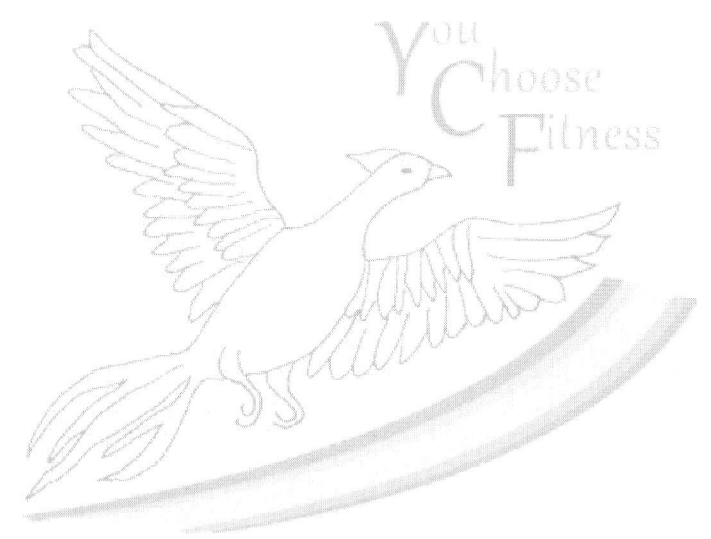

WALKING LEVELS EXPLAINED

For the walks in this book you will need to figure out your three key walking paces:

Level 1: Standard Walking Pace

A 'walk', not a stroll (but still easy).

Level 2: Walk With Purpose

A good purposeful march, arms pumping, head up, shoulders back. Imagine you have an appointment to keep.

Level 3: Power-walking

You're late for that appointment. Fast-paced march, out of your comfort zone. Real effort. Heart should be thumping!

Note: The order of these walks is completely arbitrary. You can repeat the same one or juggle them around as much as you like!

March your self-doubt into the ground

WALK ONE
STARTER FOR ……… 30?

Let's go, let's go, let's go. This walk is about you realising how much concentration it takes to walk at a pace *just slightly faster* than your natural walking pace. The slightly faster pace will be your Level 2 pace.

Your Level 3 pace is the real effort explained on page **Error! Bookmark not defined.** – standing tall, shoulders back, pumping arms and yes, breathing quite hard. You are walking **as fast as you can**!

So … Ready? The walk is divided into 5-minute intervals.

Level 2 x 1 minute, Level 1 x 4 minutes (nice and easy)
Level 2 x 2 minutes, Level 1 x 3 minutes
Level 3 x 2 minutes, Level 1 x 3 minutes = 15 minutes total

Repeat from the top = 30 minutes

> It's not about perfect.
> It's about effort.

WALK TWO
WHO FARTLEKKED?

Fartlek is part of running terminology but works perfectly well for walking, too. In running, *fartlekking* very basically means to choose a random object 50m or 100m (all loosely estimated) ahead and to sprint to it. You would repeat this exercise randomly while out on your run.

Today, you are going to *fartlek* on your walk. Your mission (should you choose to accept it) is to maintain Level 2 pace for as much of the 30 minutes as possible while incorporating EIGHT random 50m fartleks (Level 3-walking) into the time (try one every 3 minutes).

So you should walk (Level 2) for 2 minutes, for example, then choose an object about 50m away (a bus-stop, a bench, the oak tree, the street lamp, that girl talking on her phone, the bull ... No. Wait! Strike that last one! Ignore the bull! You get the idea ...). Switch to Level 3 pace – fast as you

My name is consistency. I am related to success. We should get together more often.

can – to that object. Try not to slow back down to your Level 1 (natural walking pace). You are going to try and slow down just to your Level 2!

It's quite tough. Just do your best. Take note of what you've managed. In a few weeks you can do it again and see the difference!

Repeat from the top = 30 minutes

~~I'm tired~~

~~It's too hot~~

~~It's too cold~~

~~It's raining~~

~~It's too late~~

Let's go

WALK THREE
LIKE CLOCKWORK

You'll need a watch with a secondhand or a timer of some kind for this one!

This walk is tougher than it looks so I'm going to let you choose your pace. I'll call them EASY and HARD. Your 'Easy' pace will *either* be Level 1 or Level 2. Your 'Hard' pace simply needs to be faster and tougher.

You'll need to carefully watch the timer for this one but it's easy to work out. Start at the top of every minute and do ten seconds LESS at easy pace each time and then work hard until the top of the next minute.

The Walk

Start with 5 minutes Level 1, then 5 minutes Level 2 to warm up.

Then ... a minute each of:

50 seconds EASY – 10 seconds HARD
40 seconds EASY – 20 seconds HARD

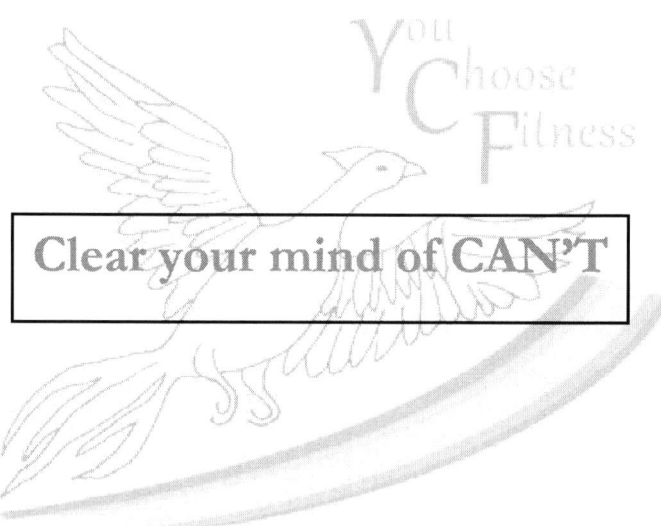

Clear your mind of CAN'T

30 seconds EASY – 30 seconds HARD
20 seconds EASY – 40 seconds HARD
10 seconds EASY – 50 seconds HARD

Rest for 1 minute

Repeat another two times

Slow walk for 3 minutes.

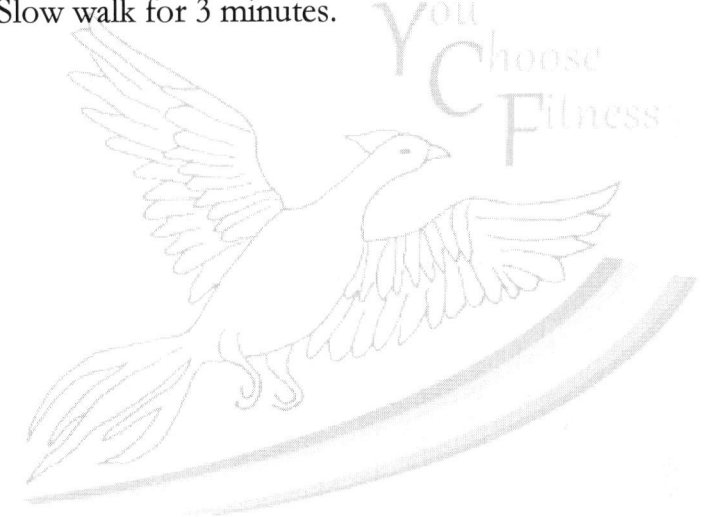

The moment you're ready to quit is usually the moment right before a miracle happens. Don't give up.

WALK FOUR
STEPPING UP A GEAR

For this 'walk' you'll need to find some steps. It can be one step or a set of steps or if you can't get outside you can use a stair. If you have trouble with balance or already find stairs a struggle, then keep this walk for another time. It is perfectly OK to hold on to the wall (outdoor steps) or the banister (indoors).

Walk at Level 1 for 5 minutes, then a full 20-25 minutes at Level 2 but today somewhere in your walk you will include EITHER:

(a) 100 steps up stairs (and down) (you only count the 'ups')

-- OR --

(b) 100 step-ups; in other words, using one step/stair, step both feet onto the step then step back down again. Step with the same leg for 50, then change the leading leg for the next 50.

If you're doing your steps or step-ups indoors you can do these at the end of a 20-minute walk.

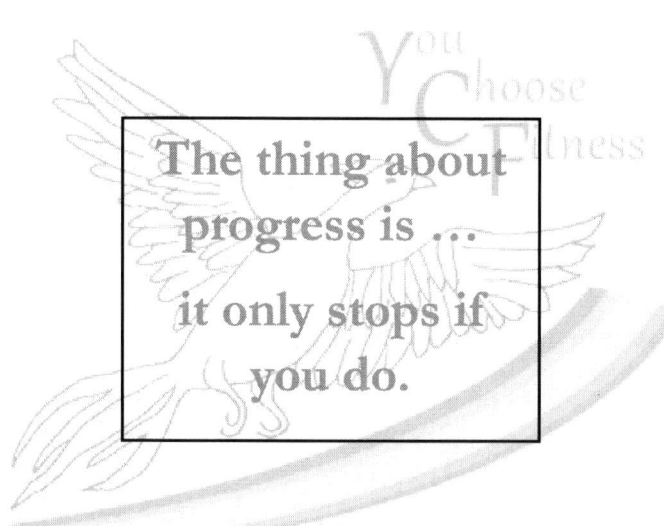

The thing about progress is …
it only stops if you do.

WALK FIVE
SIMPLE AND EFFECTIVE

One minute Level 1 then one minute Level 3

- 15 times

This one of the simplest yet most effective walks. Don't underestimate it, though. 60 seconds is not a lot of rest after 60 seconds of hard work. If you find it really tough, see how many you can manage and then try and do more next time!

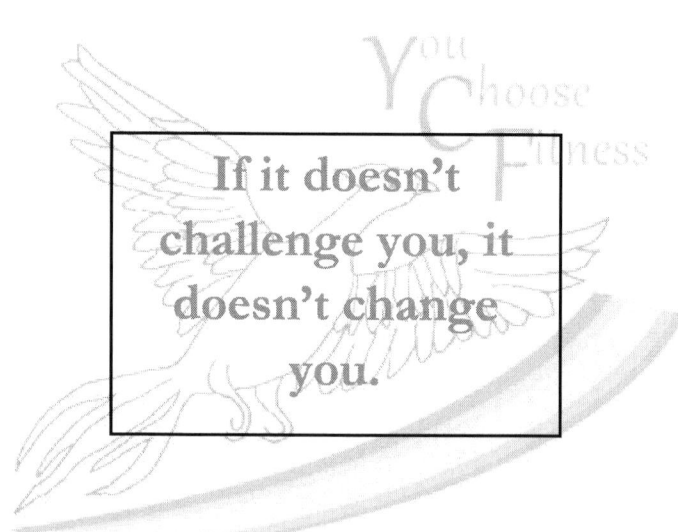

If it doesn't challenge you, it doesn't change you.

WALK SIX
TEMPO WALK

Runners do tempo runs. Walkers need to do tempo walks.

This is an out-and-back walk, not a 'loop'. This is important.

Level 1 for 5 minutes to warm up, then Level 2 for 10 minutes. Check the time on your watch and turn for home. You must walk home now in *less than* 15 minutes. In other words, your 'back' walk must be faster than your 'out'!

Pssst!! Shortcuts are not allowed!!!

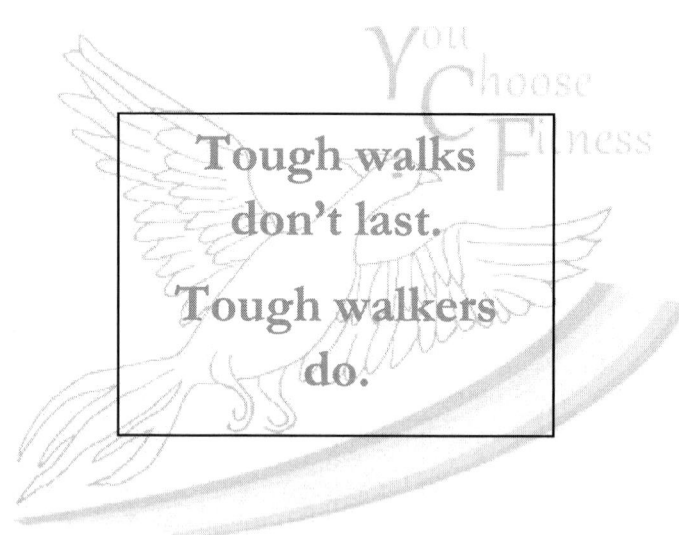

Tough walks don't last. Tough walkers do.

WALK SEVEN
HOW TO CONFUSE YOUR DOG

A watch with a secondhand or a timer of some kind would be great for this walk but is <u>not essential</u>

This walk can be tough but have fun! Challenge yourself. It's not a competition so just do what you can.

Today, you'll have two <u>interruptions</u> to your walk when you'll be moving back and forth along the same bit of path (hence confusing your dog if you're a dog-walker)!

Level 1 for 10 minutes to warm up. Now mark your starting point (wherever you happen to be) and choose a 'goal marker' about 100 metres away (house/tree/lamppost/bench …). Now time yourself from your starting point to your marker – still at Level 1. Rest 30 seconds. Walk back to your starting point at Level 2 (time should be faster). Rest 60 seconds. Once more, walk to your goal marker – but at Level 3 (fast!!)! *Note: if you don't make it faster on this last one,*

You don't have to be better than everybody else.

You just have to be better than you have been before.

rest again for a full couple of minutes and then repeat just this final 100 metres at top speed.

Level 1 for 5 minutes or so to get your breath back, then start again with your 3 x 100 metres (one at Level 1, one at Level 2, one at Level 3 – with 30 secs and 60 secs rests).

WELL DONE!

Level 1 all the way home.

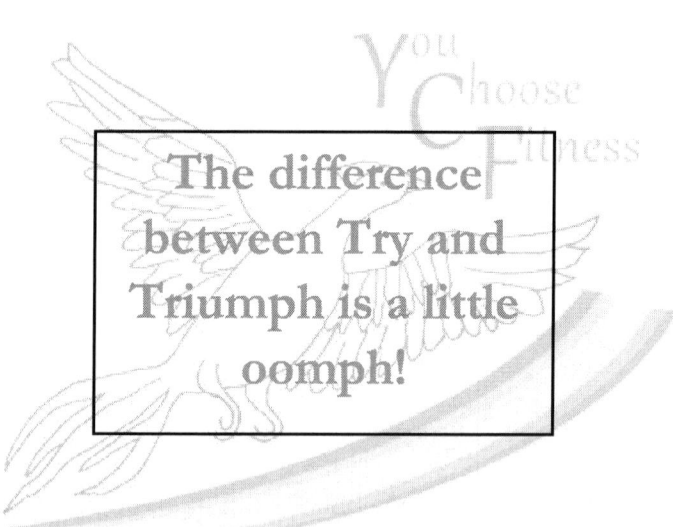

The difference between Try and Triumph is a little oomph!

WALK EIGHT
FURTHER FASTER STRONGER

Timings today give you the option to walk a little further and a little longer but this is optional! Top tip for today is to keep ALL your walking paces a little slower, so your Level 1 is almost a stroll (exceptionally), your Level 2 just a little faster than Level 1 but not excessive – and your Level 3 just a little faster again so you are out of breath but can still manage!

For the standard 30-minute walk you will go at your slowest pace Level 1 for 10 minutes, then Level 2 for 10 minutes and finish with a full 10 minutes of Level 3.

Your mission – should you choose to accept it – is to increase this to 15 minutes each (total 45 minutes).

Just do your best!

> If it's important to you, you'll find a way. If not, you'll find an excuse.

WALK NINE
POT LUCK

Very very simple walk today but a couple of decisions to make before you leave the house. The pace for the whole 30 minutes will be Level 2 so no strolling at all. However, how many 20-second Level 3 'intervals' you do within your 30 minutes will very much be pot luck! You might do lots, you might do none. Here's how it works:

YOU CHOOSE 2 or 3 (or 4) common 'markers' that you may or may not see along your walk and every time you see one of them you increase your pace to Level 3 for 20 seconds. Here are examples of some markers. You can make up yours:

Magpie or pigeon or seagull (choosing 'albatross' is cheating!!!)

White van

Somebody wearing a hat

A dog on a lead

> There's no such thing as losing. There's winning or there's learning.

A jogger

Somebody sitting on a bench

See how it works? I walk – and if I spy somebody sitting on a bench (if that's a marker I've chosen!) then I walk fast as possible at Level 3 for 20 seconds before continuing.

Being challenged in your workouts is inevitable.

Being defeated is optional.

WALK TEN
A LITTLE MORE LIKE A WORKOUT

*You can keep an eye on your watch **OR** you can guess. You just need to do everything for a minute 'or so'. You might want to scribble your mini-workout down on a piece of paper first.*

- ❖ 5 minutes Level 1 to warm up
- ❖ 5 minutes Level 2
- ❖ 5 minutes Level 3

And then ... at Level 1 ...

- ❖ 1 minute holding arms out to side and making small circles
- ❖ 1 minute standing still and marching with knees HIGH
- ❖ 1 minute Level 1 with straight arms and exaggerated swinging
- ❖ 1 minute walk on tiptoe
- ❖ 1 minute stand still and twist from side to side

Repeat these last 5 exercises

5 minutes Level 1 to cool down. **WELL DONE!**

> Success is so often a matter of hanging on after others have let go.

WHAT NEXT?
ONE STEP FURTHER ....

Never fear. If it's icy and dangerous outside – or you simply don't feel like going out - there is always something you can do indoors instead. Here are three very simple workouts you can do in the comfort of your home. Remember, it's always a good idea to challenge yourself to something different. You can do any of these workouts instead of a walk on one of the days or, even better, you can tag a workout onto the end of your walk!

Whatever you do, give it 100% and you will notice results very quickly indeed.

Note: These workouts are designed for the most reluctant exerciser and/or anyone who struggles with the common notion of 'workout'. No excuses. If you find them too easy, feel free to do them twice – or do two (one after the other)!

You don't always get what you wish for.

You get what you work for.

5 TIPS TO ENSURE THAT EVERY WORKOUT IS A SUCCESS:

1.   Gather any equipment you need (including your workout plan) before you begin. That way you won't have to keep interrupting your workout to look for things.

2.   If any of the exercises are new to you, have a little run-through before you begin so you know what you're doing. It can be very frustrating if you have to keep stopping to read instructions.

3.   Make sure you have a large glass of water standing close by. You'll need to keep sipping away throughout your session.

4.   A workout is not a competition! Don't get frustrated if you can't do an exercise for a full 60 seconds or if you struggle with any exercise. Just do as much as you can, make a note of how much you can manage and try and beat it the next time. This is a great way to measure progress! And if there's any exercise you just can't manage at all? Find something you *can* do and do that instead.

5.   Be proud that you are working towards a goal that is so so important. Your health is a gift to yourself and is worth top priority so don't 'squeeeeeze' a workout in between other 'stuff'. Make a workout appointment with yourself in your diary – just as you would a doctor's appointment (and you wouldn't miss THAT, would you?) – and allow time to get everything together beforehand and cool down and feel proud of yourself after!

10-MINUTE WORKOUT

Equipment required:

a timer/watch or clock with second hand

- ❖ 60 secs MARCH ON THE SPOT (pumping those arms)
- ❖ 60 secs HIGH KNEES (get those knees up above your waist)!
- ❖ 60 secs SUMO SQUAT PULSE (Feet wide, toes pointing outwards, bend the knees and squat (not too much). Stay low and pulse up and down. Keep bum squeezed and stay as upright as you can)
- ❖ 60 secs SWINGS (Arms by your sides, bend your knees a little and swing your arms back behind you, then swing in front and over your head, straightening your legs – as if you were going to dive off a diving board. Swing back down. Repeat without stopping.)
- ❖ 60 secs PUNCHING OUT (Feet shoulder-width apart, bring your hands up to your chin. Punch one fist straight out in front of

you. As you bring it back to your chin, punch the other fist out. Continue punching – fast as you can but making sure you straighten your arms fully each time).

REPEAT THE WHOLE FIVE MINUTES ONCE (OR TWICE IF YOU'RE LOOKING FOR MORE OF A CHALLENGE!)

15-MINUTE WORKOUT

Equipment required:
- Timer or watch/clock with second hand
- Straight-backed chair (not an armchair)
- 2 x 400g tins (tinned tomatoes or suchlike)

Do each exercise for 60 seconds and move immediately to the next

- ❖ PUNCH UP AND OUT: Stand tall and punch both hands up to the sky at the same time, then punch both hands out to the sides (shoulder height). Repeat – up and out, up and out …

- ❖ HIGH KNEES: March on the spot, raising those knees *above waist height*.

- ❖ CHAIR SQUATS: Stand in front of a chair. Without using your hands, sit down and stand up. Repeat as many times as possible. Do not lift your feet off the floor when you sit down. Your feet stay flat at all times.

- ❖ KNEE LIFTS: Sit on the chair but without touching the back. Sit tall, pull your tummy in and keep your feet flat on the floor. Raise one knee towards your chest. Pause and lower. Raise the other knee. Repeat as often as you can for 60 seconds. Do not move your body when you raise your knee – your tummy will be doing all the work.

- ❖ SMALL ARM CIRCLES: Standing OR sitting … Hold your arms out to the sides, shoulder-height. Stretch your fingers out so your arms are tense. Make tiny circles forwards and backwards. Don't drop your arms below your shoulders and keep them as straight as you can.

- ❖ BICEP CURLS: Standing OR sitting: Hold a tin/weight in each hand. With arms by your sides and palms facing forwards, glue your elbows into your sides (they must not move AT ALL!). Now raise the tin to your shoulders (slowly) by bending your elbows – then lower slowly all the way back down to your sides. Be sure that elbows do not leave your sides when bending!!

- ❖ SINGLE LEG BALANCE: Holding your weights in your hands, stand up tall, pull your tummy in, squeeze your bum and lift one foot slightly off the floor, balancing on the other. Hold this position for 60 seconds. If your balance is really good, try writing your name in front of you in the air with your other foot. **REPEAT ON THE OTHER LEG!**

❖ SUMO SQUAT AND CURLS: Stand with your feet wide apart and your toes pointing outwards (like a sumo wrestler!). Bend your knees into a squat and stay there. At the same time, holding a weight/tin in each hand, raise your arms out to the sides at shoulder height with your palms facing UP! Keeping your arms in this position, bend your elbows and bring the weights in to your shoulders, then back out – *without lowering your upper arms below your shoulders!* Repeat for 60 seconds (still holding that squat!!!)

❖ JOG ON THE SPOT: Just what it says. Jog on the spot for 60 seconds. The pace is up to you. If you struggle, then jog very lightly. If it's easy, jog faster. Pump your arms and your feet will follow!

WELL DONE!

> Don't stop when
> you're tired.
> Stop when you're
> done!

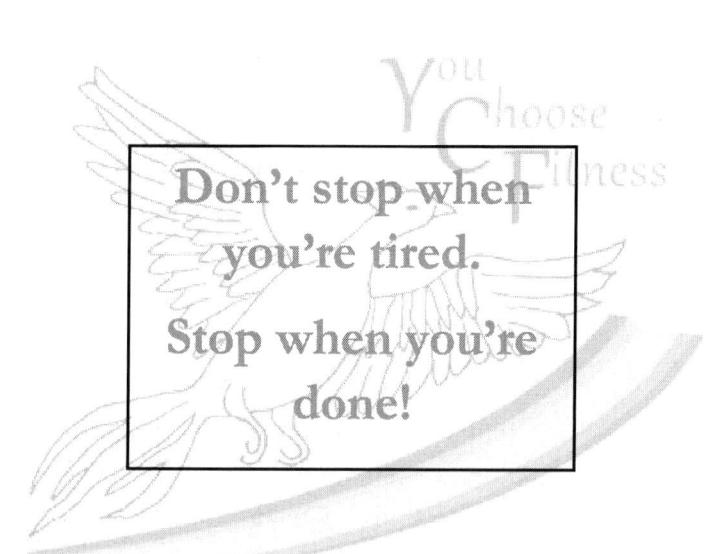

20-MINUTE WORKOUT

Equipment required:
- Timer
- A step/stair
- A straight-backed chair
- 2 weights/400g tins

WARM-UP
- ❖ 30 seconds JOG ON THE SPOT
- ❖ 30 seconds HIGH KNEES

*Do this **3 times***

MAIN WORKOUT

3 MINUTES STEP-UPS – Step both feet on and off your stair/step. Lead with one foot for 90 seconds, then change to the other foot.

REST 60 SECONDS

60 seconds SHOULDER PRESS: Hold weights at your shoulders, elbows bent and tucked in. Push up to the ceiling (palms facing) and lower back to shoulders.

60 seconds FRONT AND LATERAL RAISE: Hold weights, arms down and palms facing your thighs. Keeping your palms down, raise your straight arms in front of you, lower back to your thighs, then raise arms out to the sides (shoulder-height). Lower and raise to the front again.

60 seconds SUMO PUNCHING OUT: Feet wide apart, toes pointing outwards, lower into a squat and hold that position while you punch out, holding your weights, one arm and then the other.

REST 60 SECONDS

5 CHAIR SQUATS (sit down and stand without using hands)

4 WINDMILLS (Feet wide, arms straight out to sides (shoulder-height), bend over and twist to touch your left foot with your right hand, then twist to the other side and touch your right foot with your left hand. If you can't touch your foot, that's fine! Twist to touch your knees! It's the 'twist' that's important!. Right AND left count as 1 windmill. Try and keep your back straight.

3 OVERHEADS (Hold your arms out to the sides – shoulder-height). Raise your arms over your

head and clap your hands together. Lower your arms ONLY TO SHOULDER HEIGHT!

2 HIGH KNEES (2 each leg)

1 FORWARD BEND (try to touch your toes – or as near as!)

REPEAT THIS SEQUENCE OF FIVE EXERCISES AS MANY TIMES AS POSSIBLE FOR 5 FULL MINUTES!!

REST 60 SECONDS

60 seconds SEATED KNEE RAISES: Sitting down, sitting tall (no leaning), raise one knee to your chest and then the other.

60 seconds RUSSIAN TWIST: Sit on the edge of the chair, your TOES on the floor - and lean back! Pull in your tummy and twist to one side so you touch the side of the chair with BOTH HANDS (or as near as possible). Twist around to the other side. Make sure you are LEANING BACK!! If you find this easy, challenge yourself by taking your feet off the floor!

60 SECOND JOG ON THE SPOT or … if brave enough … JUMPING JACKS!!

WELL DONE! SUPER WORKOUT!

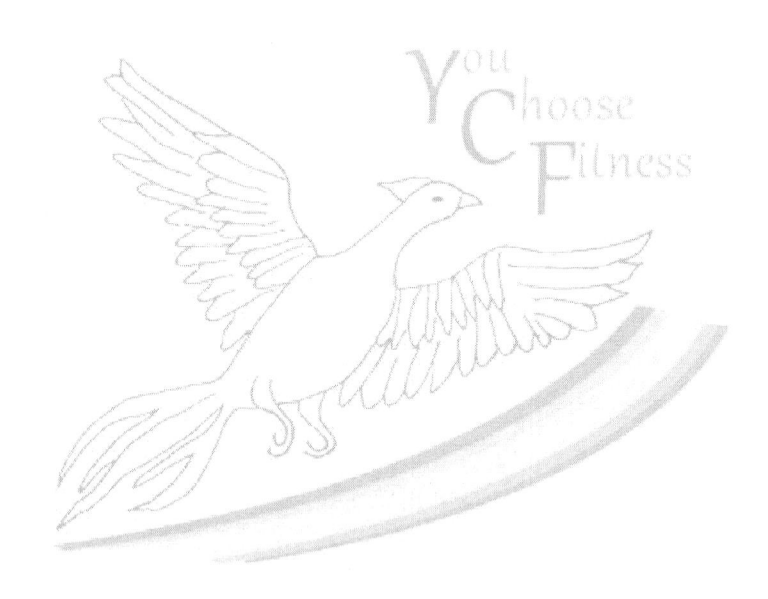

5 MOST COMMON WEIGHT LOSS ERRORS

1. Lack of variety (e.g. toast and cereal every morning for breakfast)

2. Diet sodas (worse than 'normal' sodas with even worse consequences)

3. Fat free products (any)

4. It's low-calorie so I can eat more of it! (No!)

5. Lifting weights will make me bulk up (Ladies – no! Lifting weights will kill FAT!)

No diet can do
what healthy
eating does

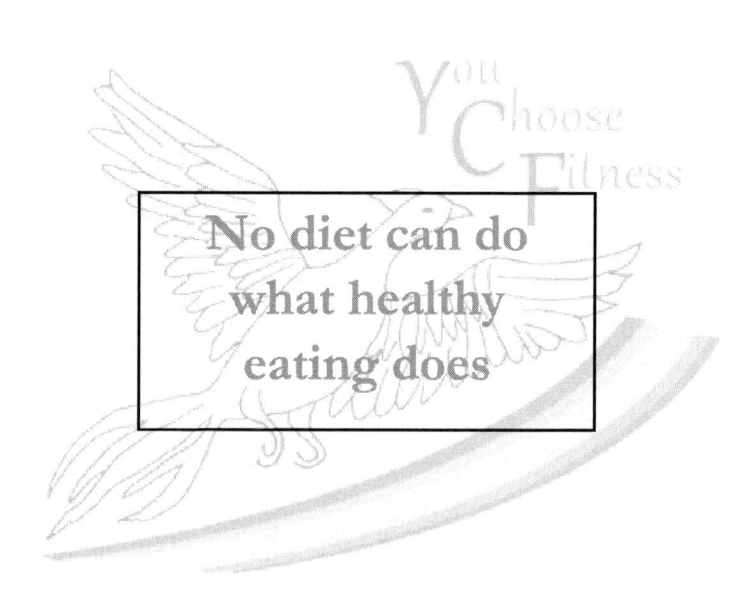

5 TOP TIPS FOR WEIGHT LOSS

1. Never repeat the same meal within a 3-day period (breakfast, lunch OR dinner)

2. Make a list before you shop and avoid any 2-for-1 or BOGOF deals

3. Eat protein with every meal

4. Eat more portions of vegetables than fruit

5. Be HONEST! If you can't possibly do without your Saturday night bottle of wine, cake/biscuits at work or Friday's takeaway, then you're not really *THAT* serious about losing weight, are you? Sort your priorities and come back determined to succeed!

Looking to kickstart your weight loss, boost your current weight loss or get off that plateau that you're stuck on?

Find out TODAY about the revolutionary and super-successful TEN DAY TURNAROUND – an online programme which has had nothing but great results. Just ten days, ten rules, 10 x ten-minute workouts for EVERY level of fitness, ten motivational texts and more!

Compatible with any other weight loss plan.

DON'T STOP THERE!

Check out the You Choose Fitness website for information on what's available

www.youchoosefitness.co.uk

Find me on Facebook: Just look for the group You Choose Fitness

http://www.facebook.com/groups/youchoosefitness

Or you can email
amanda@youchoosefitness.co.uk

Don't forget to ask about the You Choose Fitness cookbooks and meal plans.

Printed in Great Britain
by Amazon.co.uk, Ltd.,
Marston Gate.